Aronia Berries

Nature's Healing Treasure Against Chronic Disease

TERRY LEMEROND *and*
AJAY GOEL, PH.D., AGAF

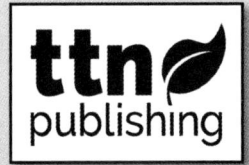

Published by:
Terry Talks Nutrition Publishing
GREEN BAY, WI

Library of Congress Cataloging-in-Publication Data is on file with the Library of Congress.

ISBN: 978-1-952507-61-8

Editor: Kathleen Barnes • www.takechargebooks.com
Cover: Jill Cashin
Interior: Gary A. Rosenberg • www.thebookcouple.com

Printed in the United States of America

10   9   8   7   6   5   4   3   2   1

Contents

CHAPTER 1

What Is Aronia?

You've probably never heard of *Aronia melanocarpa* or Aronia berries, but you may have heard of them by their common name, chokeberries. They are indeed nature's healing treasure, and they have been right under our noses since the beginning of human history.

Our ancestors were well aware of Aronia's universal healing properties, but like many pieces of ancient wisdom, much of this information has been lost.

We're here to tell you about the extraordinary healing powers of this little-known berry that can quite literally save your life.

Have you ever seen an Aronia bush? It's easy to miss the black-colored berries on a six-foot tall, unassuming shrub that may be growing unplanned in your backyard or at the edge of some woods. Its small white flowers are pretty in spring. Birds are helpful in spreading Aronia berries as seeds for new plants, and they also spread easily by suckers. A profusion of berries and orange foliage may draw your eye in the fall. The berries often persist through the winter, offering much-needed food for birds. The bush is hardy enough to withstand harsh Northern winters and is tolerant of a wide variety of soil types, moisture and acidity.

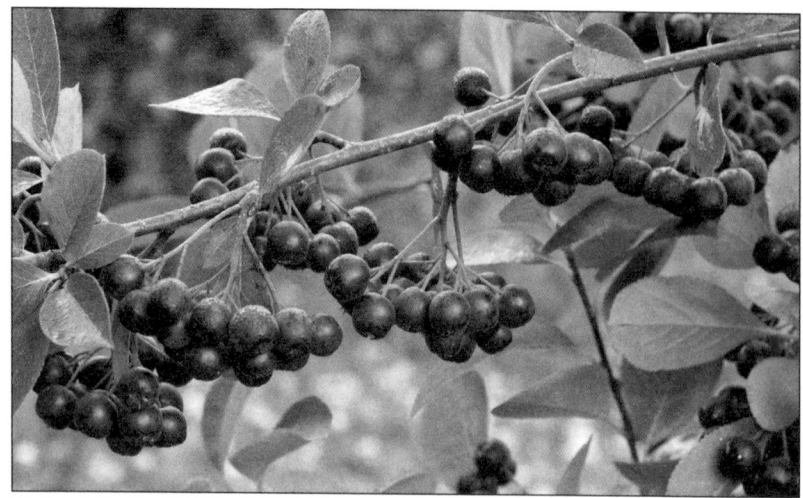

You'll find Aronia bushes growing prolifically (some say a little too energetically, but how could we have too much of a healing powerhouse?) at the edges of woodlands throughout most of North America and the northern reaches of Europe. Each bush can produce an impressive 38 pounds of berries per season.

Grab a handful of berries, and you'll probably stop after one or two because of their tart taste. In fact, the name "chokeberry" is derived from the astringent fruits that make your mouth pucker.

That's why the berries are usually processed into jams, syrups, sugar-sweetened juices and wines.

We all know the dangers of too much sugar, so today, we are fortunate enough to have naturally gathered and processed Aronia berries available as a supplement standardized to maximize their healing powers—without sugar and minus the mouth-puckering taste.

Amazing wealth

In the coming pages, we will give you the information you need about this amazing gift of nature and its impressive range of health benefits. Hopefully, you'll begin to appreciate it as a treasure unmatched in the plant world.

Aronia has extraordinary antioxidant and anti-inflammatory capabilities. We'll go into the details in the coming chapters, but for now, it's important to know two things:

1. Long-term inflammation is the underlying cause of almost every chronic disease.

2. Antioxidants can neutralize the effects of chronic inflammation, environmental toxins, and even genetic malfunctions that cause disease.

Aronia's magic

Aronia is a treasure trove of polyphenols and active antioxidant plant compounds that keep us healthy and treat and even reverse a wide range of chronic diseases.

If you're not familiar with polyphenols, antioxidants, free radicals, and chronic diseases, don't worry. In the coming chapters, we'll discuss these and other basics in depth.

For now, you just need to know that Aronia is a powerhouse against disease in ways our ancestors have known for millennia, and modern medical research is now confirming.

Aronia berries are the best choice you can make to prevent, treat, and even reverse chronic diseases and their accompanying conditions, including:

❖ **Metabolic syndrome:** This is a deadly cluster of conditions, including abdominal obesity, high blood pressure, elevated blood sugar, high triglycerides (blood fats), and low levels of HDL cholesterol that results in clogged arteries and heart disease;

❖ **Cancer:** Human studies confirm Aronia berries' effectiveness against breast, cervical, colon, liver and lung cancer, leukemia, and often fatal brain cancers called gliomas;

❖ **High blood pressure (hypertension) and unhealthy cholesterol:** These play a major role in heart disease;

❖ **Type 2 diabetes and its terrible side effects:** Heart disease, kidney disease, macular degeneration (the primary cause of blindness in the Western world), neuropathy that can lead to amputations and more are the health-destroying side effects of type 2 diabetes;

❖ **Urinary tract infections;**

❖ **Immune system enhancement:** Increased ability to fight bacterial infections and specifically the viruses that cause the flu;

❖ **All-cause mortality:** That's the technical term for protecting against death from a wide variety of chronic diseases compared to people who didn't use Aronia.

Stay with us. We'll go into all of Aronia's treasure trove of health benefits and how they work in detail in the coming chapters.

WHAT YOU NEED TO KNOW...

Aronia melanocarpa or Aronia berries, often known as chokeberries, contain a wealth of antioxidant plant compounds that prevent, treat, and even reverse chronic inflammation, a major cause of the deadliest diseases we know, especially:

❖ Cancer

❖ Heart disease

❖ Type 2 diabetes

❖ *And more.*

CHAPTER 2

Inflammation: The Good, the Bad and the Ugly

nflammation and oxidation are underlying causes of virtually every disease. The two go hand-in-hand. Stop the fires of inflammation and oxidation and you will stay healthy and slow the process of aging. It's really as simple as that.

The inflammatory cascade

Let's start with inflammation. It can be good, or it can be bad.

There are two basic types of inflammation: acute and chronic. If you've ever sprained an ankle, whacked your thumb with a hammer, been stung by a bee or gotten a cold that inflamed your airways, you have experienced acute inflammation. The redness, swelling and pain are all part of the body's natural defense system and are the initial stages of healing. Acute inflammation is an important component of the recovery process, whether from an injury or an infection.

Here's how it works: When you get a tissue injury or a viral or bacterial challenge, your body's immune system sends out white blood cells to protect you. This is the human body's natural response. Your sprained ankle, bee sting, whacked thumb or cold will hurt or cause discomfort for a while, maybe requiring a little cough medicine, pain medicine or ice, and then it heals on its own, thanks to white blood cells and the innate healing power of the human body. This is what we call a healthy inflammatory response. It's happened to every single one of us. If your immune system didn't work, you'd die the first time you got a cold or an infected splinter.

However, there's another type of inflammation that is far more insidious. Chronic inflammation can occur for a number of reasons. It may begin as acute inflammation in response to an injury or an infection, but the inflammation persists, sometimes for months and even years. This is the long-term type of inflammation that can be associated with osteoarthritis after a knee injury or a lingering cough after a bad cold, for example.

Sometimes called silent inflammation, chronic inflammation frequently has no outward signs of pain or even any symptoms at all.

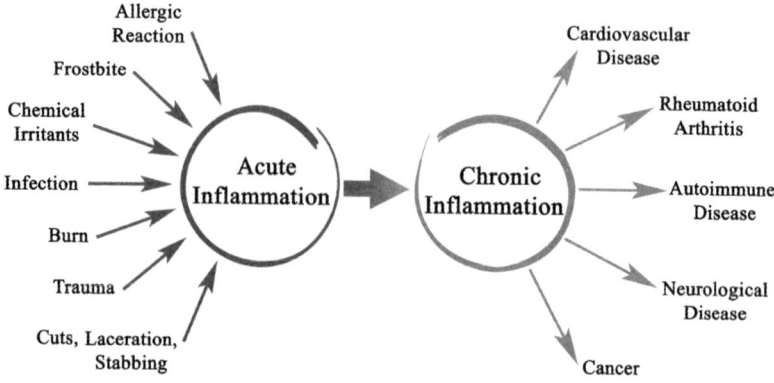

Yet, researchers for the National Institutes of Health say chronic inflammatory diseases are the most significant cause of death in the world. The World Health Organization (WHO) ranks chronic diseases as the greatest threat to human health.

Chronic inflammation is the spark that ignites disease. When chronic inflammation continues unchecked, it disrupts biological functions, damaging healthy cells and triggering inappropriate immune responses, eventually leading to DNA damage, tissue death, and internal scarring.

This insidious health destroyer may go completely unnoticed, yet it is the underlying cause of almost all chronic diseases, including obesity, cardiovascular disease, diabetes, cancer, non-alcoholic fatty liver disease, osteoarthritis, rheumatoid arthritis and other autoimmune diseases, as well as neurodegenerative diseases like Alzheimer's disease. Whether or not there is pain, these diseases and others are the direct result of inflammation. This insidious condition can damage heart and brain tissues and negatively impact virtually all body functions.

There is no doubt about it: Science is confirming over and over again that chronic inflammation is the common link that fast-tracks aging and makes us look, feel, and quite literally *be* old before our time. It can make you die before your time.

Causes

Chronic inflammation is almost always caused by lifestyle choices and by environmental factors called xenobiotics (more on that in Chapter 4), including:

❖ Eating processed and adulterated foods, especially sugar, excessive refined carbohydrates and vegetable oils

❖ Overeating

❖ Smoking

❖ Breathing polluted air

❖ Drinking municipal water

❖ Using toxic personal care products (shampoo, soap, toothpaste, makeup, deodorant and more)

❖ Toxic cleaning products

❖ Petrochemicals and gas fumes

❖ Pesticides and herbicides

❖ Living and working in toxic environments (off-gassing carpets, furniture and bedding)

The Big S

Let's add in what may be the major cause of chronic inflammation: The Big S: STRESS. Long-term unrelieved stress, like most of us experience every single day, interferes with the ability of the stress hormone cortisol to stimulate the immune system and control inflammation. For example, in a 2012 study from Carnegie Mellon University, researchers found that highly stressed people were substantially more likely to get colds when exposed to the cold virus as opposed to people whose lower stress levels promoted healthy immune function.

Beyond the increased risk of viral infections, unrelenting stress clearly opens the door and makes us vulnerable to all of those diseases we want to avoid.

We'll say this in the simplest terms possible: If you are obese or have diabetes, heart disease, Alzheimer's disease, or cancer, you have a disease triggered by chronic inflammation. These are almost always lifestyle diseases.

While you may not be able to control the air pollution in your town or the off-gassing furniture and carpet in your office (more on xenobiotics coming up), there are healthy lifestyle choices you can make that will minimize your risk of chronic inflammation and the inflammatory diseases we all want to avoid.

If you don't have these diseases yet, if you pay attention to your lifestyle choices, you can control and manage your stress levels and make significant strides toward protecting your health and preventing the inflammatory cascade that leads to serious health challenges.

While nothing will 100% guarantee that you never become obese or get heart disease, cancer, diabetes, or Alzheimer's disease, Aronia berries can give you the best life insurance policy the herbal world offers.

Warning signs you may have chronic inflammation

Some of the common signs and symptoms that can signal chronic inflammation include:

❖ General body pain and aches

❖ Elevated cholesterol

❖ Chronic fatigue and insomnia

❖ Depression, anxiety and mood disorders

❖ Gastrointestinal complications like constipation, diarrhea, and acid reflux

❖ Weight gain or weight loss

❖ Frequent infections

❖ Memory impairment

❖ Red, itchy, inflamed skin

Diagnosis of silent inflammation

How do you know if you have chronic inflammation?

There are two key blood tests that can give your doctor a profile of your levels of chronic inflammation.

The CRP (C-reactive protein) test measures how much protein your liver makes. These levels rise in response to inflammation. A CRP level between 1 and 3 mg per liter of blood often signals a low, yet chronic, level of inflammation. CRP levels over 3 mg/liter indicate serious inflammation. If there is no current acute inflammation, silent inflammation has most likely already caused one or more diseases.

A simple blood test can measure levels of fibrinogen, a protein manufactured by the liver. Often used to measure bleeding disorders, lately, fibrinogen has also been used to measure chronic inflammation. Normal fibrinogen levels are 200 to 300 mg/dl.

WHAT YOU NEED TO KNOW...

Inflammation is the body's natural defense against an injury. It assists in the healing process by bringing infection-fighting white blood cells to the area, usually causing swelling and heat. Long-term inflammation may not produce any symptoms at all. It can occur for a number of reasons:

❖ Prolonged elevated inflammation that was once acute

❖ Exposure to toxic substances, including environmental pollutants

❖ Poor lifestyle choices

Chronic inflammation can cause a host of chronic diseases, including:

❖ Several types of cancer

❖ Heart disease, including hypertension and high cholesterol

❖ Type 2 diabetes

❖ Alzheimer's disease

❖ Gastrointestinal disorders

❖ Depression and anxiety

❖ Osteoarthritis

❖ Non-alcoholic fatty liver disease

❖ Rheumatoid arthritis and a variety of autoimmune diseases

CHAPTER 3

Oxidation: Inflammation's Evil Twin

We need to breathe oxygen to stay alive, so it's a good thing, right? Sure, it is, but too much of a good thing can become a bad thing.

When you breathe in oxygen, the oxygen molecules (oxidants) are normally converted into water by your cells. But sometimes, that process goes awry, particularly as we age. Then that water causes problems. Have you ever noticed rust on the bumper of your car? Think of oxidation as "rust" on vital cells that make up every system in your body. It disrupts cellular function on virtually every level, leaving you vulnerable to the chronic diseases we've been presenting in this book.

Oxidative stress

That oxygen-generated "rust" gives birth to disease-causing free radical oxygen molecules (usually called "free radicals") that impair your body's ability to process fats and proteins and can even alter DNA. This disease-causing condition, called oxidative stress, can happen for many reasons, including:

❖ Emotional stress (we've heard that one before, haven't we?)

❖ Chronic inflammation

❖ Toxic exposure

❖ Glycation (impaired sugar metabolism)

❖ Poor lifestyle choices

Oxidative stress is the second branch in the disease-causing process. At least 90% of modern-day diseases are caused by oxidative stress and inflammation.

Cell Deterioration

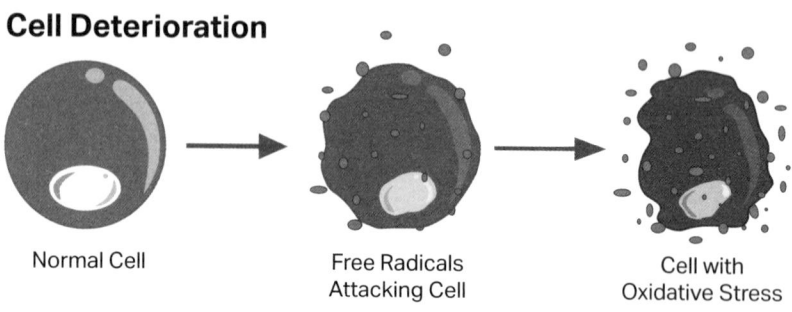

Normal Cell   Free Radicals Attacking Cell   Cell with Oxidative Stress

Oxidative stress and inflammation go hand-in-hand. They feed off each other in a downward spiraling cycle. You'll remember about inflammation from Chapter 2. When inflammation and oxidative stress join up like Bonnie and Clyde, they can cause immense damage to your health, opening the door to cellular aging and genetic deterioration, as well as to diseases of aging, including cancer, heart disease, diabetes, liver disease, dementia, and Alzheimer's disease.

What are antioxidants?

Harvard scientists give us a simple explanation: "Antioxidants neutralize free radicals by giving up some of their own electrons. In making this sacrifice, they act as a natural "off" switch for the free radicals. This helps break a chain reaction that can affect other molecules in the cell and other cells in the body."

Science has repeatedly confirmed that a diet rich in antioxidants derived mainly from fruits, vegetables and beverages such as tea, coffee, olive oil or wine is essential to the prevention of premature aging, cardiovascular disease, cancer and virtually all the diseases of aging.

Think of your overall health as a bank account. Simple dietary and exercise choices can have an impressive positive effect on your "bank" balance.

Add Aronia berries to your daily regimen for a treasure trove of antioxidant compounds, especially polyphenols, flavonoids including carotenes, lutein, anthocyanins and proanthocyanidins, and your health "bank" account balance will grow exponentially. Aronia berries have the highest concentration of the powerful anthocyanins of all berries.

Of course, you don't have to be over 50 to benefit from these healthy choices. The earlier in life you access these nutrient treasures, the richer your health "bank" account will be over your lifetime.

Consider this: Aronia berries score over 16,000 on the ORAC (Oxygen Radical Absorbance Capacity), a USDA scale that measures a food's ability to eliminate free radicals.

Aronia berries are off the chart, eclipsing antioxidant powerhouses like cranberries, blackberries, raspberries and blueberries.

As you can see from the ORAC chart that follows, the 16,000+ rating for Aronia is triple that of blueberries.

Until recently, this was a reasonably useless comparison since few of us would eat the 100-gram (about 3.5-ounce) standardized serving of Aronia berries because of their mouth-puckering properties. Now that Aronia is available as a palatable supplement, its disease-busting wealth is easily accessible to all of us.

One of those concentrated Aronia powders has been found to contain a mind-boggling 52,000 ORAC units per tablespoon!

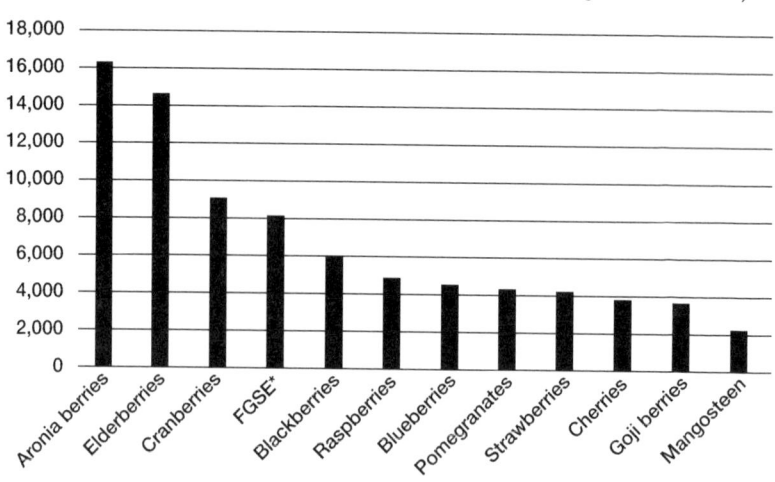

ORAC Berry Comparison of Fresh Berries
(ORAC values from USDA comparison are based upon 100g of fresh berries)

*FGSE = French grape seed extract   Table courtesy of USDA

Note: Chart does not include the Acai berry because a powder was used in the study rather than a fresh berry.

Why is this important? Research proves that consuming foods with high ORAC values can raise the antioxidant levels in your blood by as much as 20%.

Most of us take in 3,000 to 5,000 ORAC units on a good day, but scientists are now projecting that we need 10,000 to 12,000 ORAC units a day to significantly affect antioxidant levels and provide protection against all forms of free radical damage.

More Aronia treasure

Without descending too far into science-speak, let us say that the human body can produce five types of free radicals: hydroxyl, peroxyl, peroxynitrite, singlet oxygen and superoxide. Each can cause a different type of damage.

So, we're looking for a nutrient that will target all five. Aronia berries provide that unique protection and so much more, considering what we already know about Aronia's anti-inflammatory powers.

You'll see in the next chapter that a third aspect of Aronia's treasure makes it the best possible choice you can make for a long, healthy life.

WHAT YOU NEED TO KNOW...

Aronia berries combine their anti-inflammatory powers with those of one of nature's most potent antioxidants to prevent and reverse the chronic diseases that can shorten your life:

❖ Disease-causing free radical oxygen molecules are the major culprits in chronic diseases, including cancer, heart disease, type 2 diabetes, liver disease and dementia.

❖ Aronia berries, with their incredibly high antioxidant rating, neutralize free radicals and protect against all of these diseases.

❖ Aronia is now available as a supplement, offering all of the disease-fighting properties of chokeberries without the tart taste.

CHAPTER 4

Xenobiotics: Our Toxic World

Xeno what? We're not surprised if you've never heard of them, but we can guarantee they are dangerous to your life and your health.

From the Greek words "xeno," meaning foreign, and "bios," meaning "life," xenobiotics are substances foreign to life. These artificial chemicals, not found in nature, are sometimes called "forever chemicals" because they are nearly indestructible.

Even the tiniest exposure in the parts per *quadrillion* can cause harm.

These toxic chemicals are everywhere: in our air, water, and soil, in environmental pollutants, food additives, hydrocarbons, cosmetic additives, flavoring and fragrances, hydrocarbons from vehicle exhausts, pesticides and herbicides. They are also in our non-stick cookware, waterproof clothing and food packaging. Some of them are even found in prescription drugs, including some chemotherapy drugs used to treat cancer.

Forever and everywhere

Xenobiotics surround us everywhere we go. They're in the air we breathe, the water we drink, the food we eat, the clothes we wear, the beds we sleep on, our phones, televisions, computers, and even our furniture. Heck, they're even in the aspirin you take for a headache and the plastic wrap on your veggie tray. Forever chemicals have even altered soil composition, reducing microbial components of soil and altering the nutrients in our food crops.

It's impossible to completely avoid them, but there are ways we can neutralize some of their health-destroying effects. Stay with us.

The human body is always working to excrete toxic substances. When you take xenobiotic chemicals—or any toxins—into your body, your liver, kidneys and lungs will process them and eliminate them as fast as possible through feces, bile and exhalation. Sometimes that's just not enough.

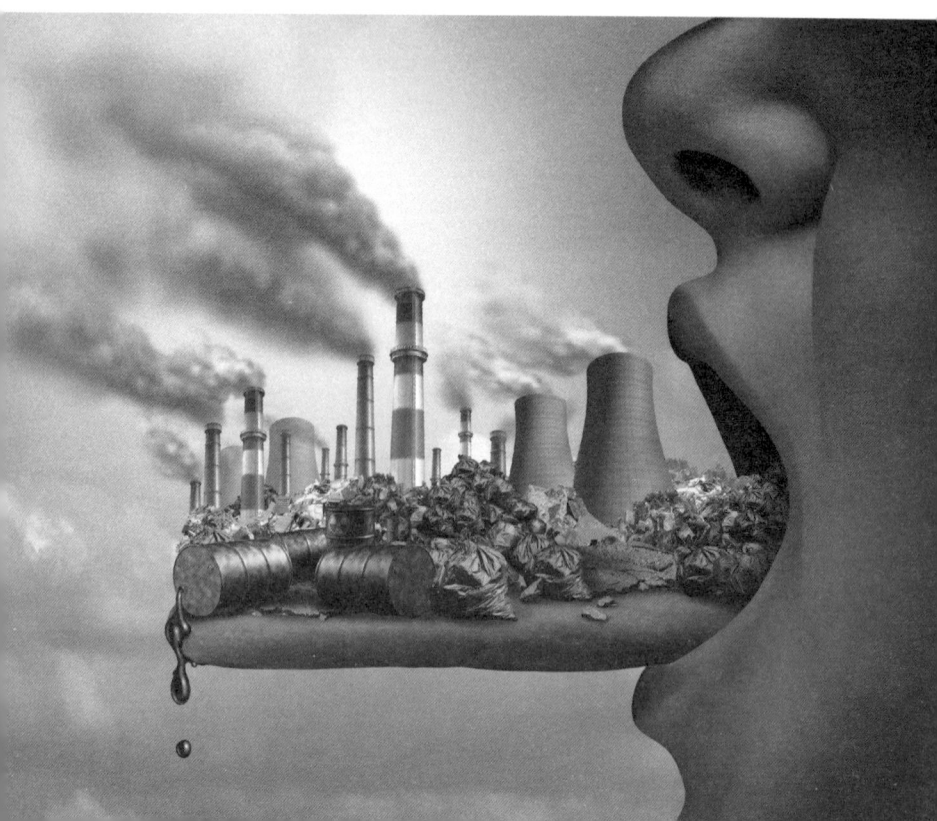

What harm can xenobiotics cause?

Many xenobiotics are endocrine disruptors implicated in the rising levels of obesity, type 2 diabetes and a host of metabolic disorders that affect virtually every system in mammals and probably other life forms. When hormonal messengers and cellular reproduction are disrupted, quite literally, all hell breaks loose in the human body.

Xenobiotics can cause dysbiosis (yeast overgrowth in the digestive system that can cause imbalances in virtually all bodily systems), congenital disabilities, reproductive disorders, developmental delays in children, several types of cancer, liver disease, obesity, type 2 diabetes, heart disease, Alzheimer's disease and many more illnesses, the mechanics of which are not fully understood.

We also need to look at the effects of xenobiotics on other species. A just-published British study on European hedgehogs shows widespread poisoning caused primarily by constant exposure to pesticides and herbicides. Are these little hedgehogs the canaries in the coal mine? Probably.

We like to think of our newborn babies as new and pure, but that is hardly the case in today's world.

Science has now shown us that xenobiotic substances can pass through the placental barrier between a woman and her child and into the baby's bloodstream. In at least 40 studies conducted over the past six years, researchers confirm that toxic chemicals were found in every single cord blood sample taken from newborns.

How terrible to think that these tiny humans are already susceptible to a host of diseases before they even take their first breath! It's even worse to think of chronic diseases that were once the province of middle and old age, like type 2 diabetes, that are now becoming common in the teen years.

We think it is abundantly clear that the omnipresence of xenobiotics is a culprit in our deteriorating collective health.

The worst of the worst

A pivotal 2011 study from the National Institutes of Health confirmed that 39 million (yes, 39 MILLION!) artificial chemicals were commercially available 13 years before this writing.

Clearly, we're not going to name them all, but there are a few that are the major culprits:

PFAS (per- and poly-fluoroalkyl substances) are probably the most ubiquitous and most harmful. According to the US Environmental Protection Agency, they are used to make products that resist heat, oil, stains, grease and water. They are long lasting and break down very slowly, sometimes over hundreds and even thousands of years.

Phthalates keep plastics flexible. They are used in a wide range of products, from nail polish and garden hoses to shoes, safety glass additives, printing inks, and rocket fuels. They can cause birth defects and reproductive harm.

"In the USA, more than 340 million pounds of phthalates are consumed every year and cause potential health and environmental risks. Phthalates can easily leach into food, water, and other products applied directly to the human body. Some dairy products, fish, seafood and oils are found to have a high level of phthalates," according to researchers in a 2021 paper.

POPs (persistent organochlorine pollutants) are pesticides that have concentrated in the food chain and have now reached alarming levels in the human population. They are endocrine disruptors and are known to cause cancer, allergies, central nervous system damage, immune system impairment and developmental delays in children.

Pesticides (DBCP, malathion, atrazine) widely used in agriculture harm the soil ecosystem and wash into waterways, spreading their harmful effects. Atrazine has recently been definitively tied to breast cancer. Malathion, mainly used to control mosquitoes, has been shown to cause cancer, neurodevelopmental harm, and reproductive toxicity.

What you can do

Clearly, we can't avoid breathing, drinking water or eating, at least not for very long, so here are some simple ways to reduce xenobiotic exposure and avoid the health havoc they can cause you and your family.

Here's a seven-point To-Do list:

1. **Eat a healthy diet:** This means eating organic as much as possible, with a wealth of fruits, vegetables, healthy fats, whole grains and legumes and lean, organically produced meat and fish. Cruciferous vegetables, including broccoli, cauliflower and cabbage have been shown to help neutralize and eliminate toxins. Other healthy

toxin-defining foods include berries, apples, garlic, tomatoes, olive oil and ginger.

2. **Healthy supplements:** Probiotics can help protect your gut and keep toxins from gaining a foothold or even reverse the damage xenobiotics may have already caused. Here's where Aronia comes in. Several studies now point to Aronia as an effective way to neutralize the damage caused by xenobiotics as well as fight inflammation and oxidation. More about that in Chapter 5.

3. **Eliminate plastic:** We know that's a tall order. It may even be impossible to fully implement. No, we're not telling you to scrub your home of everything plastic and dump it all in the landfill. That will only contribute to the toxic circle. Think twice about buying anything plastic, especially single-use items like food wrappers, bottles (even if they're recyclable), toys and food storage containers.

4. **Wash your produce:** Almost all produce, even oranges and watermelons that have a rind you won't eat, has some level of pesticide contamination. Rinsing under cold water for 30 seconds will remove contaminants in most foods.

5. **Filter your water:** A whole house filter is optimal since you absorb toxins from municipal water even when you shower. If that's not possible, at least use a reverse osmosis filter on your drinking and cooking water.

6. **Clean out your bathroom cabinet:** Shampoos, soaps, cosmetics, toothpaste, skin care products and just about everything else in your bathroom cabinet and cleaning supplies (and in your garden supplies) contains xenobiotics. Become an avid label reader to find healthy alternatives.

7. **Redecorate wisely:** If you're considering buying furniture, painting your walls, or remodeling your kitchen, be very aware of VOCs (very toxic volatile organic compounds). You'll find them in some paint, new furniture, new carpets and rugs and fiberboard (MDF) used in furniture and cabinets. There are low- or no-VOC products available. If you have no choice, do your remodeling in the warm months so you can keep windows open and stay outside as much as possible for at least a week and consider buying older furniture made entirely of solid wood.

WHAT YOU NEED TO KNOW...

Xenobiotics are toxic chemicals that are universally present in our environment and have devastating health effects on adults, infants, and even fetuses.

✤ Many are connected with plastics, pesticides (including herbicides and insecticides) and even pharmaceutical drugs.

✤ Xenobiotics are often endocrine disruptors, meaning they affect every system in the human body and can cause reproductive harm, congenital disabilities, developmental delay, cancer, obesity, type 2 diabetes, neurological disorders like Alzheimer's disease, liver disease, and many more.

✤ To neutralize the effects of xenobiotics, eat a healthy, clean diet, wash your produce, eliminate single-use plastic as much as possible, get rid of toxin-filled personal care products, cosmetics, cleaning supplies and garden supplies, and find healthy alternatives.

✤ Probiotics, cruciferous vegetables, and Aronia berries can help neutralize the toxic effects of xenobiotics.

(For more information, see the article "Xenobiotics in Health and Disease: The Two Sides of a Coin: A Clinician's Perspective" at https://juniperpublishers.com/oajt/OAJT. MS.ID.555641.php)

CHAPTER 5

A Home Run!

We don't mean to be too "inside baseball" (pun intended), but Aronia is a home run for your health! It hits all three major disease-causing bases we've talked about in the opening chapters of this book and then some:

❖ Inflammation

❖ Oxidation

❖ Xenobiotics

For the sake of brevity, let's lump these three together and call them IOX since we know that when one of the three exists, it's highly likely that the other two are also present. The three IOX dangers combined pose a serious threat to your health.

When those three threats can be contained and even overcome, the result can be vibrant health and a long life. Aronia is the batter that hits that home run.

A plant that can overcome these three health-destroying conditions is a rare treasure, indeed. When we find two such plant treasures, we've hit the health jackpot! (More about the second plant treasure in Chapter 10.)

It's a home run for your health.

Aronia is one of less than a handful of botanicals scientifically proven to address all three simultaneously.

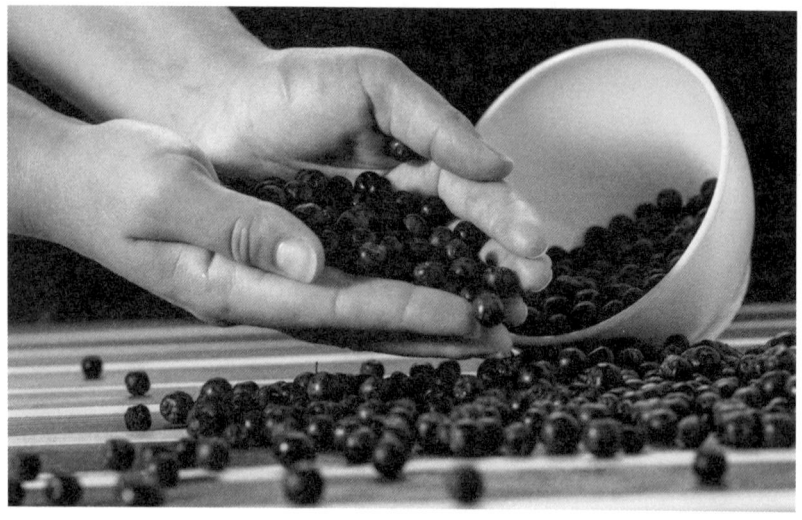

The proof?

One Polish study lauded Aronia berries as "a very rich source of numerous substances exerting a beneficial impact on health."

In our opinion, that's an understatement, especially when it comes to Aronia's wealth of nutrients that combat IOX.

Inflammation

We'll take a deeper dive into Aronia's heart healthy properties in the coming chapters, but it's important here to point out Aronia's superstar anti-inflammatory chops are largely displayed in its proven heart-protective benefits.

A 2012 study published in the *European Journal of Nutrition* attributes Aronia's unique health protecting abilities to dietary polyphenols, which are super anti-inflammatories and antioxidants. We've pointed out that anti-inflammatory and antioxidant properties are difficult to separate.

Let's start with polyphenols, super antioxidants found in abundance in Aronia berries, including anthocyanins, proanthocyanidins, quercetin, rutin, chlorogenic acid, and epicatechin.

A growing body of research confirms that eating foods rich in polyphenols like Aronia helps regulate metabolism, protect against weight gain and chronic disease, and minimize out-of-control cell division that can lead to most types of cancer.

Polish researchers found that Aronia had a higher polyphenol content than resveratrol, the red grape-based substance that has sometimes been called the key to longevity.

They said, "*Aronia melanocarpa* fruits are one of the richest plant sources of phenolic substances shown to have anti-inflammatory, antitumor, antioxidative, and antiplatelet activities."

Oxidation

Remember the ORAC index from Chapter 3 that shows Aronia literally off the scale for its antioxidant power to knock out disease-causing free radicals? That's the key to understanding how Aronia berries can help get your body back on the road to health.

There are five major free radical oxygen molecules: hydroxyl, peroxyl, peroxynitrite, singlet oxygen and superoxide. Aronia seems to have a laser focus to knock out these most dangerous free radicals.

The same Polish scientists also found that an extract of Aronia berries increased levels of glutathione, a super antioxidant produced in the liver, perhaps the most potent antioxidant in our cells. It's the gatekeeper, if you will, blocking the entry of disease-causing oxidants, inflammatory markers and xenobiotics into our cells.

Glutathione protects the immune system, aids in building and repairing tissue, improves insulin sensitivity in people with type 2 diabetes, slows and even reverses cancer progression, and can also reactivate (regenerate) depleted antioxidants—especially vitamins C and E—so they can resume neutralizing free radicals.

Xenobiotics

Glutathione has a unique ability to help sweep toxic metals out of the system, including mercury in batteries, disinfectants, fluorescent light bulbs, fish and seafood, cadmium in some manufacturing processes, and cigarette smoke. Aronia has been shown to activate the body's natural glutathione defense system.

A 2016 Polish study confirms Aronia berries' ability to help us neutralize the effects of xenobiotic toxins.

"...only a little attention has been paid to the possibility of their use to counteract the adverse health effects of exposure to xenobiotics. That is why in this review article, the main interest has been focused on the possibility of using chokeberries to protect against unfavorable health effects caused by the action of substances to which humans may be exposed environmentally and/or occupationally."

Their conclusion in the study: "The available experimental data indicate that not only the fruit but also the leaves of *Aronia melanocarpa* and their products may be effective means for prevention and treatment of the effects of toxic action of some xenobiotics in humans; however, further studies on this subject are necessary."

Another study confirmed that treatment with Aronia berries improved bone strength in women who had bone loss due to toxic cadmium exposure.

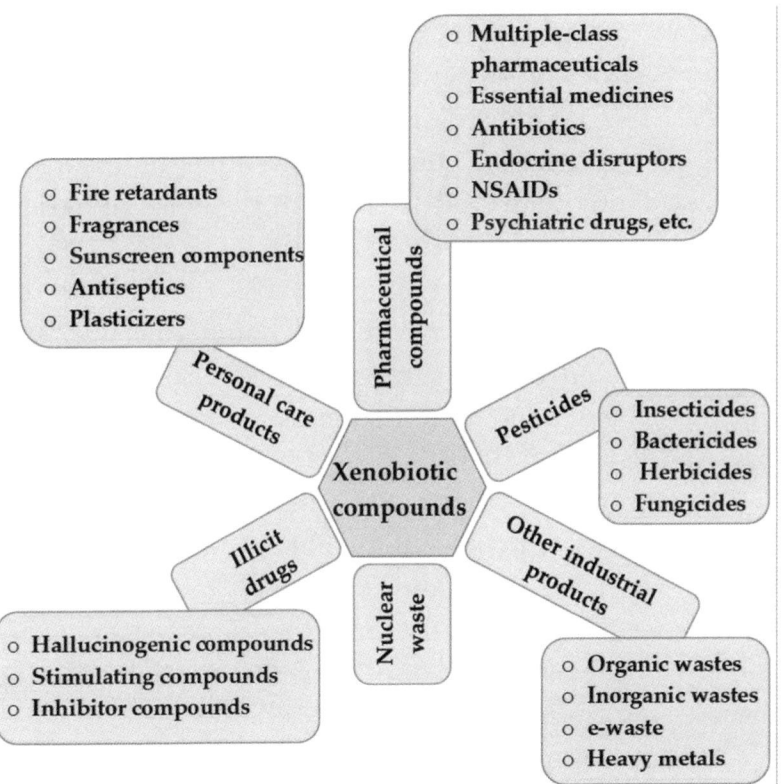

Plus epigenetics

We want to introduce a fairly new term—epigenetics—that is directly related to xenobiotics.

Epigenetics is the study of how your lifestyle choices and your environment specifically affect the way your genes work. These outside (non-genetic) changes can "turn on" or "turn off" genes that control, for example, how your body responds to a cancer-causing substance in the environment, such as tobacco smoke.

Epigenetics is a relatively new field of science. Simply put, your diet and lifestyle, your caloric intake (most of us eat entirely too much!), your environment and your exposure to toxins determine how your genes work and dictate whether those genes are well-behaved or whether they go rogue. Epigenetics explains the continuously changing behavior of your gene structure and, for our purposes here, your body's genes in response to various environments. One element of epigenetics is DNA methylation, which governs how genes behave.

Dr. Goel's research has uncovered numerous ways epigenetics influences genes that promote or control cancer, but this type of gene malfunction can affect virtually any gene in the human body.

When you don't eat a healthy diet or exercise regularly and are exposed to toxins—remember those xenobiotics?—that is everywhere, including the air we must all breathe and the water we must all drink, cancer-preventing genes can go to sleep on the job or become hyperactive, allowing diseases to take a foothold.

As you age and grow, it is natural that some genes may

get turned off—or go to sleep—as a consequence of eating habits, exercise regimens, and toxic environmental stresses. Other genes that encourage uncontrolled cell growth may get turned on, thus promoting cancer growth. Those that prevent cancer in several ways may get turned off.

Unlike the small risk for hereditary cancers, cancer-related genes that are epigenetically controlled and are directly related to lifestyle choices are responsible for more than 95% of all cancers.

Certain substances can stimulate those genes to wake up or calm down. You probably won't be surprised to learn that Aronia berries hold a rare place in the plant world because of their ability to regulate those rogue genes and get them back to their normal state. We'll have more about that in Chapter 8.

In a 2021 study by a consortium of researchers from several countries, including the United States, confirmed Aronia's ability to direct genes to revert to their original purposes in overweight women with heart disease. A German study confirmed that drinking an Aronia juice extract for just four weeks helped repair frayed or broke DNA strands in healthy men.

WHAT YOU NEED TO KNOW...

Aronia is one of the few substances scientifically confirmed to cover three essential bases in human health. It is:

- ❖ Anti-inflammatory

- ❖ Antioxidant

- ❖ Anti-xenobiotic

That means that Aronia addresses virtually all of the chronic diseases usually related to aging, including heart disease, cancer, obesity, type 2 diabetes, Alzheimer's disease, and many more.

CHAPTER 6

Cancer

D r. Goel has spent his life researching how various plant medicines can prevent, treat and even cure cancer. While his research at Baylor University and most recently at the City of Hope has focused on colorectal cancer, supporting research confirms that Aronia and other botanicals can have profoundly positive effects on a wide variety of cancers.

This research solidifies Aronia as Mother Nature's treasure: a powerhouse way to address IOX (inflammation, oxidation and xenobiotics), the conditions that are the underlying cause of most chronic diseases, especially cancer.

We all know someone who has had cancer. We know its far-reaching and devastating effects. Maybe some of us have had the disease.

Even those lucky enough to "beat" cancer often fall victim to a recurrence or a spread of cancer cells months or even years later.

Even as science is gaining ground in the fight against some forms of cancer, other deadlier types of cancer are taking their place. In fact, cancer, the second most significant cause of death in the United States, is rapidly gaining ground against heart disease, the Number 1 killer of Americans.

It's a huge advance that metastatic breast cancer is now treated as a chronic disease rather than a terminal, debilitating illness. Patients with many skin, breast, and prostate cancers may live long and productive lives, an unthinkable possibility even a few years ago. However, lung, colorectal, and pancreatic cancers are on the rise, especially among younger people.

Based upon estimates by various national organizations, within the next 10 to 20 years, the number of cancer deaths in the United States will almost triple.

These are grim facts, but needless to say, it's time to take this threat *very* seriously.

We've all heard that cancer "runs in families." With the exception of some very specific genetic anomalies, like the BRCA gene that causes breast and ovarian cancer, the vast majority of cancers are the direct results of xenobiotics, including geographic location that might be linked to

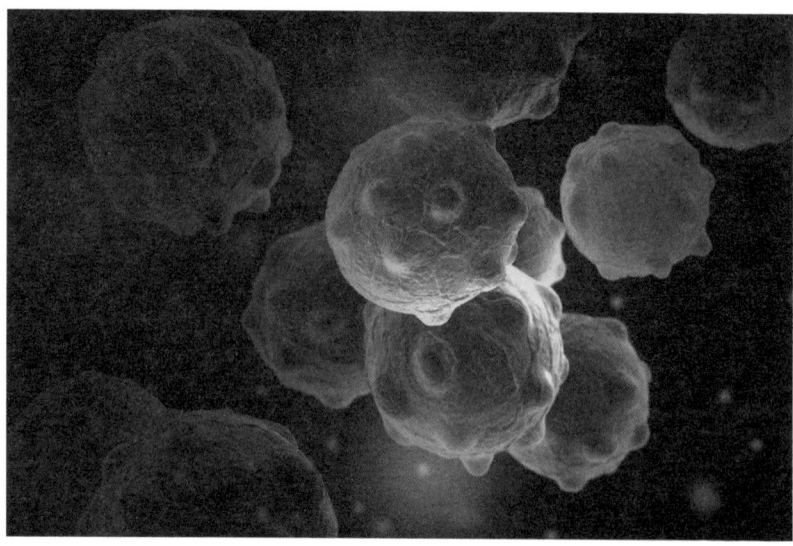

toxic exposure and family dietary and lifestyle choices that leave us vulnerable.

It seems that virtually all cancers start when, as Harvard researchers said in a paper, "a few stem cells that have lost their genetic marbles, so to speak . . ."

Remember from Chapters 2, 3, and 4 that Aronia is a treasure house of polyphenols, the precise nutrients that combat almost all types of disease?

Without oversimplifying the process by which cancer starts, grows and spreads, let's start with a few processes that are common to virtually every type of cancer:

1. **Cell proliferation:** This is the wild and uncontrolled cell growth that produces exponentially larger numbers of cells than natural cell division, in which each cell replaces itself with just one exact identical twin. When that process goes awry, cancer begins. With most types of cancer, that means tumors begin to form. Myeloma and leukemia are exceptions because blood cancers do not form tumors, although they are the product of wild cell proliferation as well.

2. **Apoptosis:** This goes hand-in-hand with cell proliferation. Apoptosis is the natural life cycle in which all cells live and die. When apoptosis is disrupted, cells begin the out-of-control division that leads to cancer.

3. **Cancer stem cells:** If you have had cancer or you know someone who has had it, you know that cancer often returns, sometimes years after a "cancer-free" pronouncement by doctors. That's because treatment-resistant cancer stem cells can "sleep" for years before

entering the bloodstream and emerging in some other part of the body. This is slightly different from metastasis since hard-to-kill cancer stem cells occur in the early stages of the disease and can survive even the most aggressive drug therapy and reappear, usually in another part of the body.

4. **Metastasis:** This is the spread of cancer through the bloodstream and/or the lymphatic system from its primary location (for example, the breast, the colon or the lung) to another location (for example, the brain or liver), sometimes years after the initial cancer diagnosis.

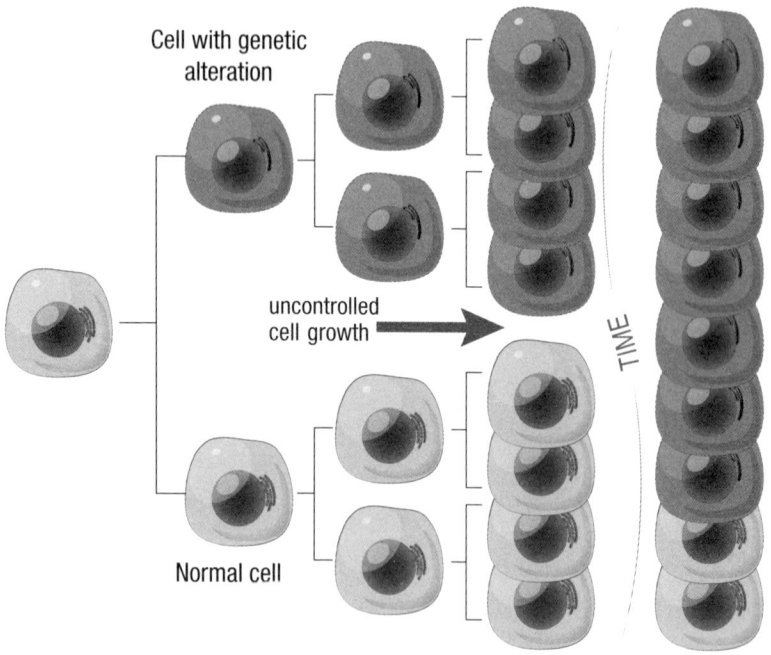

Cancerous cells: continuous division of cells that take over healthy cells, and do not submit to senescence or apoptosis (normal cell death).

Aronia: The anti-cancer treasure

By now, it probably won't surprise you that Aronia berries and their abundance of polyphenols have been scientifically validated to attack cancer in important ways.

Cell proliferation and apoptosis

A pivotal 2022 study from Ohio State cites previous research confirming Aronia's effectiveness against human breast, cervical, colon, glioblastoma, liver, leukemia and lung cancer. The study credits the polyphenols procyanidin, anthocyanin, cyanidin glycosides and caffeic and chlorogenic acids for stopping the wild cell division that launches most cancers.

Specifically, the Ohio State study credits Aronia berries for selectively targeting colon cancer cells while protecting healthy colon cells, a major advance since cancer treatment often damages healthy cells. They also found that Aronia extracts have a unique ability to help overcome cancer cells' resistance to a variety of cancer treatments, making chemotherapy drugs and radiation more effective in lower dosages.

British researchers confirm that Aronia reinstates apoptosis, restoring the natural life cycle of cells and their replacement with identical healthy cells.

Overcoming chemoresistance

The Ohio State study also confirms that gemcitabine, a chemotherapy drug, proved more effective against usually deadly pancreatic cancer when combined with Aronia berries, and Italian researchers found that the chlorogenic acid that is abundant in Aronia can work synergistically to improve the effectiveness of doxorubicin, a chemo drug used to treat several types of cancer.

Metastasis and stem cell proliferation

Korean researchers tracked Aronia's ability to knock out breast cancer stem cells and French research shows that Aronia treatment stops wild cell division, induces apoptosis and kills embryonic cancer stem cells.

What's the magic anticancer ingredient?

Researchers at California State University credit Aronia's wealth of polyphenols, anthocyanins and phenolic acids with a unique ability to slow or even stop the out-of-control cell growth characteristic of virtually all types of cancer. Their study on colon cancer cell lines called *Aronia melanocarpa* a "potent anticancer agent." Researchers noted that the black chokeberries (*Aronia melanocarpa*), compared with red and purple varieties, were the most effective anticancer agents.

A Polish study confirms the benefits of Aronia and explains that the antioxidant power of these berries can stop DNA damage in invasive breast cancer before and after surgery and/or chemotherapy.

Quercetin in Aronia has also been confirmed as a major component rare in the plant world, preventing metastasis and eliminating cancer stem cells. Particular types of polyphenols, called anthocyanins, are also major players in Aronia's effectiveness against cancer.

Dr. Goel's research

Dr. Goel's team at the City of Hope has spent years researching Aronia's anticancer benefits, especially as they relate to colorectal cancer. They attribute Aronia's anticancer value to a variety of polyphenols, concluding that it might be especially helpful in advanced cancers when surgery is not an option.

The team's studies found that an Aronia berry extract slowed cell proliferation, cellular survival and invasion of the cells, as well as inducing cell death in the cancer cells and stopping metastasis. The findings concluded that Aronia berry extract acts as a safe and effective complementary and integrative medicine approach against colorectal cancer.

WHAT YOU NEED TO KNOW . . .

Aronia berry extracts have been scientifically validated as valuable ways of preventing, treating, and even stopping the recurrence of a wide variety of types of cancer by:

❖ Stopping out-of-control cell growth that eventually leads to cancer;

❖ Re-establishing the natural order of cellular life and death;

❖ Stopping the birth of cancer stem cells that can survive even the most aggressive cancer drug treatments;

❖ Enhancing the effectiveness of pharmaceutical cancer treatment by weakening cancer cells and protecting healthy cells;

❖ Stopping metastasis, the spread of cancer to other parts of the body.

CHAPTER 7

Heart Protection

Globally, there are more than 500 million people with heart disease. That's about 16% of the world population.

Heart disease has been the leading cause of death in the United States since 1950. Nearly 700,000 people of all races and ethnicities die of heart disease every year in the US, accounting for one in every 5 deaths.

We all know someone who has heart disease. It's probably fair to say that many of us know someone who has died of heart disease. If that doesn't grab your attention, it should.

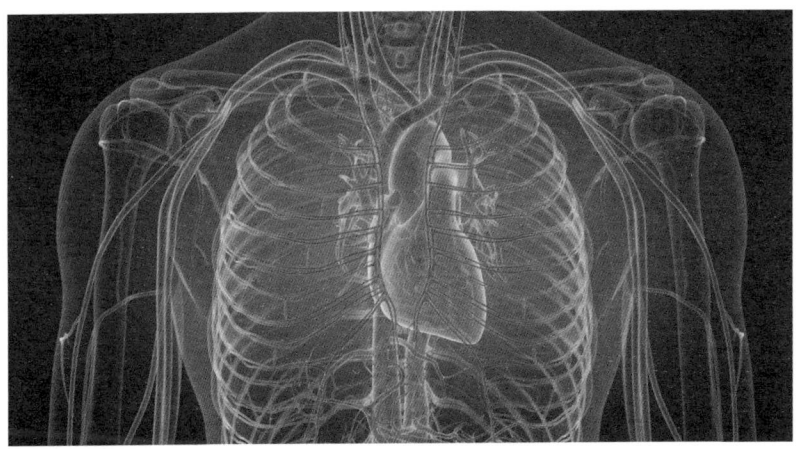

We could go on and on with statistics, but there is one take-home message: Heart disease is extremely serious. We all need to do whatever we can to prevent it, address it and reverse it. This is an important message for those already in the throes of high blood pressure, cholesterol issues and hardening of the arteries (atherosclerosis). It's lifesaving information if you've already had a heart attack (myocardial infarction) or a stroke. It's a warning for those of us who have managed to avoid these issues for now.

Dysbiosis, inflammation, and heart disease

Did you know that the state of your gut bacteria (microbiome) can directly affect your heart?

When the bacterial population becomes unbalanced (the medical term is dysbiosis), a broad range of toxic bacteria can penetrate the intestinal wall and cause problems elsewhere in the body, including the heart, triggering a broad range of heart problems.

You've probably heard of the risk factors for heart disease: aging, obesity, type 2 diabetes, smoking, secondhand smoke, unhealthy diet and a sedentary lifestyle. Those exact risk factors are also closely associated with dysbiosis, especially by allowing dangerous bacteria to circulate through the body and find new homes in the cardiovascular system.

That imbalance of gut bacteria also alters immune function and increases inflammation.

We've heard about inflammation before. Here it is again: Cardiovascular disease is an inflammatory disease.

Plant medicines like Aronia help control inflammation, rein in the wide-ranging damage of dysbiosis, and reduce the risk of heart disease.

Aronia protects your heart

That's one of many places where Aronia, nature's treasure, comes into the picture.

Recent British studies confirm that Aronia berries help protect against heart disease, and they attribute that benefit to Aronia's positive influences on the gut microbiomes.

In a 2019 study published by the prestigious *American Journal of Clinical Nutrition*, researchers attributed the "rich sources of polyphenols" in Aronia berries and extract to the improvement in arterial elasticity (meaning the blood vessels relaxed, lowering blood pressure) in as little as 2 hours after consuming Aronia and continuing through the 12 weeks their male subjects participated in the study.

That research was confirmed in another British study in 2022 that included women in the study group.

Those researchers concluded, "... the present findings suggest that daily consumption of Aronia berry extract led to improvement in arterial function in healthy middle-aged people with a concomitant and related increase in potentially health-promoting (gut) bacteria..."

Aronia's other heart-healthy gifts

Danish researchers looked at 17 published studies on Aronia and made some interesting conclusions:

"*Aronia melanocarpa* is rich in polyphenols and

compared to berries of other plants, its berries have the highest concentrations. Its berries have the highest concentrations compared to those of other plants. Due to its high polyphenol content, *Aronia melanocarpa* may be effective in treatment and prevention of cardiometabolic diseases and related risk factors. Interestingly, no studies have reported adverse effects of *Aronia melanocarpa* consumption."

Researchers at Tennessee's Franklin School of Integrative Health Sciences concluded that Aronia is an effective way to lower blood pressure and cholesterol in people over 50.

Here's another encouraging result from Serbian researchers: For former smokers who are at high risk of heart disease even though they have stopped smoking, long-term Aronia supplements helped improve protection against heart disease.

Antioxidant

Other studies confirm Aronia's antioxidant effects, resulting in improved cholesterol profiles and lower blood pressure levels. They attribute these benefits to two abundant polyphenols in Aronia berries: chlorogenic acid and quercetin.

Ohio State University researchers who reviewed several Aronia studies concluded, "Aronia juice may prevent the occurrence of cardiovascular disease, and the phenolic compounds that possess potent antioxidant activity may be the main active components involved."

In addition, several studies confirm that Aronia is an excellent way to control blood sugars in type 2 diabetes.

This is an important part of Aronia's disease-busting activity since type 2 diabetes and heart disease often go hand in hand.

Finally, Polish research suggests that Aronia can help prevent and treat xenobiotic-caused liver damage due to high blood fats, which are also a factor in heart disease.

That's another home run for Aronia when it comes to the prevention and treatment of heart disease, even among those who have multiple risk factors, including obesity, smoking and type 2 diabetes.

WHAT YOU NEED TO KNOW...

Research confirms that regular consumption of Aronia berries or their extracts can protect against heart disease in a variety of ways:

❖ Lowering blood pressure

❖ Reducing and preventing oxidation of LDL cholesterol while increasing beneficial HDL cholesterol

❖ Relaxing stiffened blood vessels

❖ Helping clear fatty deposits in the arteries

❖ Reducing inflammation, a major factor in heart disease

❖ Combating free radical damage and disease-causing oxidative stress

❖ Neutralizing damage caused by disease-causing environmental toxins called xenobiotics

CHAPTER 8

Anti-Aging and Much More

We're sure you're already deeply impressed with Aronia's vast healing powers. We certainly are.

But we're not done yet.

There is a host of other things Aronia can do. Some are related to the deadly triad of IOX (inflammation, oxidation and xenobiotics), while others are not so clearly connected. All are powerful promoters of good health and long life.

That's the beauty of botanicals. Unlike pharmaceuticals that are almost always formulated by extracting one or two elements from the immensely complex components of plant medicine, Mother Nature has created a perfect balance of what we need to heal a broad range of illnesses and what we need to protect the parts of us that are already healthy. Mother Nature always knows best!

Perhaps Aronia's greatest gift is the gift of a long life. It goes without saying that preventing and controlling IOX and its direct influence on diabetes, heart disease, cancer and other chronic diseases of aging would contribute to a longer, healthier life. However, studies show that people taking Aronia were far less likely to die of any cause than those who did not take it.

Korean researchers who tested Aronia on fruit flies, which are often used for lifespan research because their lifespans are short and it's fairly easy to document an extended lifespan, say it might even extend our lives.

Researchers noted that Aronia's ability to neutralize free radical oxygen molecules makes this plant antioxidant treasure a way to slow the aging process.

They found that Aronia supplementation extended the fruit flies' lifespan by an impressive 10%. Yes, we know we're not fruit flies, and sometimes those results don't apply to humans, but they are still significant.

Russian researchers found an even more powerful anti-aging effect from Aronia, calling it a "geroprotector." This means it affects the root causes of aging (inflammation, oxidation and xenobiotics) and age-related diseases.

Researchers credited Aronia's abundance of polyphenols for "The geroprotective properties . . include the following effects:

1. lifespan extension in model organisms,

2. amelioration of the biomarkers of aging,

3. low toxicity,

4. minimal risk for adverse events,

5. improvement of the quality of life,

6. evolutionarily conserved mechanisms,

7. reproducibility on different models,

8. prevention of age-associated diseases,

9. increased resistance to environmental stress factors."

That's enough for us to take Aronia daily, almost like a superpower multi-vitamin and recommend it to our family members as well.

Here are some of Aronia's other treasures:

Anti-diabetic and anti-obesity: Obesity and type 2 diabetes almost always go hand in hand. The Centers for Disease Control and Prevention estimates that 89% of Americans with insulin-resistant diabetes are overweight or obese.

Alarmingly, people who are obese are three times more likely to develop type 2 diabetes and the host of deadly side effects that accompany it, including heart disease, kidney disease, blindness and nerve damage that can lead to amputations.

One of the most interesting recent studies was published in the *Journal of Medicinal Food* in 2021 and concluded that Aronia berry extract lessened the inflammatory effects of eating a high-fat/high-sugar diet. Researchers credit Aronia's anthocyanin, a polyphenol, for reducing inflammation, neutralizing free radicals and helping control blood sugar.

Research on type 2 diabetes (using an animal model) showed that Aronia extract reduces insulin resistance, helps control blood sugars, promotes weight loss and reduces the risk of fat accumulation in the arteries.

In humans, Bulgarian researchers found that Aronia significantly lowered fasting blood sugars and helped control blood sugars over three months, reducing HbA1c (blood sugars over the past three months) levels from 9.39 to 7.39. That's a substantial improvement!

Anti-obesity: Obesity causes its own health issues separate from diabetes.

One pivotal Japanese study confirmed Aronia's glucose-controlling benefits and added something truly important: Aronia helps reduce belly fat. Abdominal obesity is enormously dangerous and can in itself cause heart disease, stroke, dementia and liver problems, as well as type 2 diabetes.

Worse yet, belly fat can nearly double the risk of dying prematurely, according to a study of more than 350,000 European men and women published in *The New England Journal of Medicine.*

Serbian researchers found that Aronia supplementation reduced waist circumference in postmenopausal women who were morbidly obese (more than 80 pounds above ideal body weight), a demographic that finds it very difficult to reduce belly fat.

Immune system enhancement: Aronia seems to work in a different way to combat infections, whether they are viral (like COVID-19) or bacterial (like a urinary tract infection).

Part of Aronia's immune system enhancement comes from the well-known benefits of its high vitamin C content and a plethora of vitamins and minerals, including B vitamins, magnesium, iron and zinc.

Norwegian researchers who studied elderly nursing home residents who were particularly susceptible to urinary tract infections (UTIs) found that they are vulnerable to Aronia's natural antibiotic effects. They credited the cyanin polyphenols with reducing UTIs by 55% in people who took Aronia for three months.

Austrian research confirms Aronia's value as an antibiotic and verifies impressive improvements in the body's ability to fight infections of all types. For example, researchers found that Aronia reduced viral load against the flu and SARS-CoV-2 by as much as 80%, an impressive finding in preventing these infectious diseases and controlling their spread.

Researchers applauded polyphenols again: "These anti-influenza properties of Aronia were attributed to two constituents, ellagic acid, and myricetin . . . Based on these results, we suggest that Aronia is a valuable source for antiviral agents and that (polyphenols) ellagic acid and myricetin have potential as influenza therapeutics."

Neuroprotective: Aronia has the unique ability to cross the blood-brain barrier, opening the door to protecting the brain from dementia and Alzheimer's disease, Parkinson's disease, and a variety of other neurodegenerative disorders.

Aronia is also a key element in protecting neurons (brain and nervous system cells) from deteriorating or dying due to oxidative stress.

A 2022 animal study found that Aronia improves memory and protects brain cells from the beta-amyloid plaques characteristic of Alzheimer's disease. The antioxidant anthocyanin polyphenols found in abundance in Aronia are credited with improving memory and other neuroprotective benefits.

Researchers at the University of Nebraska determined that Aronia extracts protect brain cells from death or damage caused by inflammation and free radical oxygen molecules. Quite specifically, they found that Aronia's xenobiotic benefits protect brain cells that have been damaged by exposure to the herbicide paraquat, which is known to cause Parkinson's disease.

Dutch research confirms that six months of Aronia extract supplement slowed cognitive decline in people who were at high risk of mental deterioration and worsening neurological diseases.

Other studies have confirmed Aronia's protective effects against the "normal" cognitive decline associated with aging, especially with overweight men over 60.

And Serbian scientists found that those magical anthocyanins relieved anxiety and stress in lab animals.

Liver protective (hepatoprotective): Fibrosis, the accumulation of scar tissue in the liver, is caused by inflammation. It is often linked to alcoholism, chronic hepatitis, and non-alcoholic fatty liver disease.

Korean researchers found that Aronia helps reverse non-alcoholic fatty liver disease and improves the liver's ability to process fats.

Aronia can also reverse fibrosis and help restore the balanced ecosystem of gut microbes that are commonly unbalanced in people with liver disease.

Metal detoxification: Polish researchers found Aronia protects the body against cadmium poisoning caused by cigarette smoke, exposure to batteries, lead, and a variety of foods grown in contaminated soil. The human body has great difficulty removing this xenobiotic toxic heavy metal, so it generally accumulates in the kidneys, where it can cause cancer.

Several studies now confirm that Aronia helps activate the body's natural antioxidant defenses to chelate (eliminate) toxic metals like cadmium while protecting the body's vital zinc and copper balances at moderate doses.

When we add all of these factors up, Aronia offers a way to prevent, treat and even reverse the diseases of aging, offering us a healthier, longer life.

WHAT YOU NEED TO KNOW . . .

Aronia has impressive capabilities to fight a number of communicable and non-communicable diseases. Most of its treasure still lies in the polyphenols that fight inflammation, oxidation and xenobiotics, thereby leading to longer lives in lab animals and possibly in humans.

Aronia has been scientifically validated as a preventive and treatment for:

❖ Obesity

❖ Diabetes

❖ Immune system dysfunction and bacterial and viral infections

❖ Alzheimer's disease

❖ Parkinson's disease

❖ Cognitive decline

❖ Depression and anxiety

❖ Liver disease

❖ Exposure to toxic heavy metals

CHAPTER 9

Add in French Grape Seed Extract

What happens if we marry Aronia, the superpower that combats the triple threat of inflammation, oxidation, and xenobiotics (IOX), with another plant superpower that does the same?

We have an anti-aging combo that cannot be beat. It provides what our bodies need to prevent, treat, and even cure the diseases caused by that triple threat.

You've probably heard the term "synergy," which means the combination of two things is greater than the simple sum of the individual parts. In this case, the two substances enhance one another's already formidable healing powers.

So, if we add French grape seed extract (FGSE) to Aronia, we find synergistic healing that cannot be matched in the plant world.

What is FGSE?

French grape seed comes from the royalty of grapes. Think of French wine, and you'll quickly get the idea: There is nothing better!

Our ancestors loved wine fermented from grapes. Today's science has confirmed the health benefits of wine, many of which are derived from the seeds themselves. Concentrating those life-giving and even life-extending benefits into grape seed extract makes FGSE a potent tool that should be added to your medicine cabinet, whether you are suffering from one of the many diseases of aging or if, like all of us, you want to avoid them.

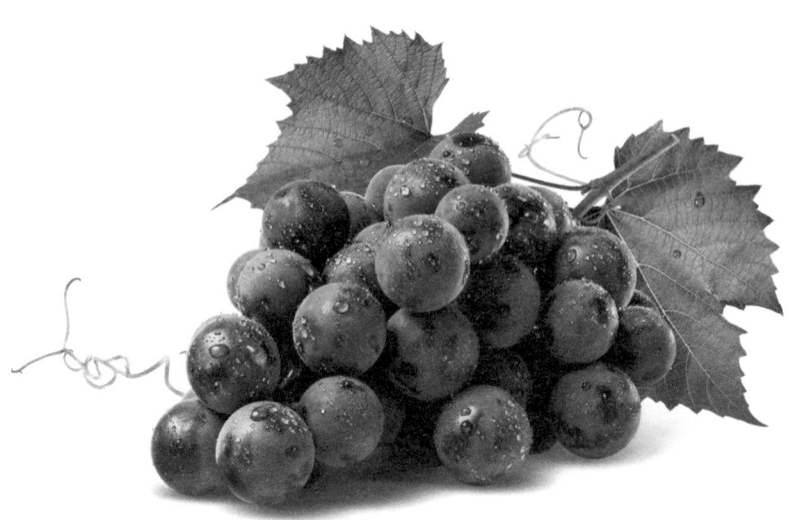

Polyphenols again!

A major part of FGSE's power comes from polyphenols. Does that surprise you? Probably not if you've read this book from the start.

These polyphenols, with the tongue-twisting name oligomeric proanthocyanidins (OPCs), are concentrated at extraordinary levels in grape seeds, hence their healing power.

OPCs are right at the top of the list, with Aronia as the most potent antioxidant known to science.

The antioxidant levels in grape seed extract are so high that they are quite literally off the scale. Antioxidant ability is reported as the ORAC value (oxygen racial absorbance capacity), a measure of a food's free-radical-fighting capabilities. The ORAC value of low molecular weight French grape seed extract is an astounding 21,000 per gram!

This power pair eclipses other antioxidant powerhouses like cranberries, blackberries, raspberries and blueberries.

There are only a handful of botanicals known today that can achieve these remarkable healing feats:

❖ Reduce inflammation, an underlying factor in many chronic diseases

❖ Treat and even cure cancer by attacking it in several ways

❖ Lower blood pressure

❖ Strengthen and relax blood vessel walls

❖ Lower cholesterol and triglycerides

❖ Control blood sugars

❖ Assist in weight control

❖ Protect brain cells

❖ Protect memory by helping create neural pathways as alternative pathways to transmit information

Does this list sound familiar? It's a list of FGSE's health benefits, almost identical to the list of Aronia's treasure house of health benefits. But here's the main point: It's not a duplication. Combining the two offers a healing gold mine.

Put the two together, and you have a dream team of benefits attributable mostly to polyphenols, but they work in slightly different ways. Think of it as covering all the bases to get us to that home run for our health if we combine Aronia with French grape seed extract.

FGSE and cancer

Dr. Goel has spent his career researching plant medicines, particularly their effects on cancer. FGSE has generated huge excitement from Dr. Goel and his team at the City of Hope as well as in the scientific community for the following scientifically validated reasons:

❖ Stop inflammation, an underlying cause of cancer

❖ Stop oxidative stress

❖ Stop the negative effects of environmental toxins

❖ Protect smokers

❖ Reduce tumor size

❖ Stop cells from becoming cancerous

❖ Stop the formation of blood vessels that feed cancerous tumors (angiogenesis)

❖ Signal cancerous cells to commit suicide (apoptosis)

❖ Target cancer stem cells, the major reason why cancers spread (metastasis)

❖ Awaken sleeping genes that stop the growth of cancerous cells or slow down genes that are telling cells to reproduce wildly (epigenetics)

❖ Overcome the body's natural rejection of chemotherapy drugs over time (chemoresistance)

❖ Works synergistically with other natural treatments, including Aronia.

If you recall the ways Aronia combats cancer and all of these diseases from the earlier chapters in this book, you'll recognize the overlaps and the potential for exponential plant power against the deadliest diseases known to science.

We both feel very strongly that the answer to addressing heart disease, cancer, diabetes, and dementia and finding the pathway to a long and healthy life starts with Aronia, French grape seed extract and a handful of other plant medicines that are Mother Nature's gift to give us the long, healthy lives that are our birthright.

WHAT YOU NEED TO KNOW . . .

From head to toe, the antioxidant power of Aronia and grape seed can keep your body healthy and strong, from preventing dementia to reducing the risk of nerve damage in hands and feet.

❖ Both botanicals offer a wealth of disease-busting polyphenols that overcome inflammation, oxidation and xenobiotics, the underlying causes of almost all chronic diseases.

❖ Both have been deeply scientifically validated to overcome several aspects of heart disease, including high blood pressure, congestive heart failure and blocked arteries that can lead to heart attacks and strokes.

❖ Both have also been shown to combat cancer in several novel ways.

❖ The variety of polyphenols between the two "fills in the gaps" in disease prevention. Aronia is rich in several types of cyanins and FGSE in oligomeric proanthocyanidins that complement and even escalate one another's healing powers.

CHAPTER 10

How to Use It

From Terry Lemerond:

Our ancestors must have been more challenged than we are since they freely availed themselves of the health benefits of Aronia despite its tart taste, similar to a dry wine. They had good reason to call these berries "chokeberries!"

We can be thankful that all those benefits are painlessly available today in supplement form!

Let's take a look at the perennial question: How do you find the right product?

I often get that question. It's almost always followed by another question: "How do I know this contains the actual botanical I'm looking for?"

And then: "How do I know it's safe and not laced with toxins?"

Those are all excellent questions.

There are several supplements available on the market, and you'll need to do a little investigation to find the right one:

Sometimes, the final product contains little or no actual Aronia. Sometimes, the berries are contaminated during the harvesting and storage process. Sometimes, they are even adulterated with other substances, some as benign as other plant products and sometimes with prescription drugs, about which you'd have no knowledge.

Look for Aronia that has been processed, tested and standardized into capsules for consistent levels of polyphenols. This is the only way I know of to be certain you are getting a clean product that will do what you need it to.

Standardization. Look for a product that is lab tested and, for purity and quality, standardized to 40% polyphenols for the concentrated, consistent delivery of Aronia's wealth of health benefits.

Since we've examined the synergistic value of French grape seed extract (FGSE) and Aronia, it's worth looking for a product that combines the two. How convenient! For the highest absorbability, the FGSE content of your supplement should be 80% absorbable, low molecular weight tannin-free oligomeric proanthocyanidins (OPCs), and 99% polyphenols.

Those little capsules reassure me that I am getting exactly what I want and need every single day. It's much more convenient, especially if you travel often, like I do.

Another tip: Quality companies will always include their contact information on their packaging.

All you need is one capsule standardized to 200 mg daily. However, if you are dealing with any of the serious health conditions covered in this book, some experts suggest taking up to 5 doses daily on a regular schedule.

As always, you know your body best, you should consider other supplements you might be taking for potential interactions. Neither Aronia nor FGSE have any serious side effects, but they can cause mild gastrointestinal problems when you first start taking them. That's why it's best to consult your healthcare practitioner.

If, as is often the case, your healthcare practitioner is not familiar with Aronia or FGSE, please copy the next chapter and offer it as documentation of their potential value in preventing and treating a broad range of diseases and even extending your life.

WHAT YOU NEED TO KNOW . . .

Aronia and FGSE make a great partnership to combat the deadliest diseases associated with aging. Animal models confirm they can extend lifespans.

❖ Look for an Aronia product that is lab-tested for purity and quality, standardized to 40% polyphenols for the concentrated, consistent delivery of the botanical's wealth of health benefits.

❖ Look for a French grape seed extract product that contains 80% absorbable low molecular weight tannin-free oligomeric proanthocyanidins (OPCs) and 99% polyphenols for the highest absorbability.

❖ For even more potent effects and convenience, look for a prepared combination of Aronia and French grape seed extract.

CHAPTER 11

For Healthcare Professionals

From Dr. Ajay Goel:

Most authors are protective of their work and prohibit copying and distributing book contents unless the books are sold or paid a royalty.

This section of this book is very different. This information is so important that my co-author, Terry Lemerond, and I want to see it distributed far and wide. At least as far as this chapter goes, we are unconcerned about copyright.

We also know that doctors and other healthcare practitioners are very busy. They are very unlikely to read an entire book, even though, like this book, it may contain some information that could save lives or help improve the quality of life of their patients. We understand that doctors are frequently skeptical about natural formulations and, if they haven't conducted their own research investigations on a subject, they are inclined to steer their patients away from them, even though these formulations might be lifesaving.

We've created this short chapter, a synopsis of the most important elements of this book. We encourage anyone to copy it freely and pass it on.

Dear Doctor,

Your patient has given you a copy of this chapter with my blessings and permission. My publisher and I have given it to the public domain so that the vital information it contains on the value of *Aronia melanocarpa* (also known as black chokeberry) can be broadly circulated.

I have spent more than 20 years researching the preventive and treatment properties of botanicals, primarily for cancer prevention and treatment, in my previous tenure at Baylor University and my current tenure at the City of Hope.

I've published more than 400 studies on various aspects of health and cancer in high-impact journals around the world, including numerous studies emphasizing the health benefits of complementary and alternative medicine and treatments based on Traditional Chinese Medicine and Ayurvedic tradition.

I urge you to take a few minutes to read this section and consider how Aronia's scientifically validated unique properties can prevent and treat humankind's most deadly diseases.

—*Ajay Goel, Ph.D., M.S., City of Hope Professor and Chair, Department of Molecular Diagnostics and Experimental Therapeutics; Associate Director of Basic Science, Comprehensive Cancer Center (formerly Baylor University's Center for Gastrointestinal Research and the Center for Epigenetics, Cancer Prevention and Cancer Genomics)*

Aronia melanocarpa, commonly known as black chokeberry, has unique and substantial anti-inflammatory, antioxidant, and anti-xenobiotic properties that make it one of medicine's most powerful botanical tools to prevent chronic diseases of aging and a variety of infectious diseases.

Science has long confirmed that inflammation, oxidation and xenobiotics are the underlying causes of cancer, heart disease, type 2 diabetes, neurological diseases such as Alzheimer's disease and many more.

The credit goes to an abundance of polyphenols found in Aronia, including anthocyanins, procyanidins, flavonols, and hydroxycinnamic acids, which are unparalleled among botanicals. In fact, Aronia has been rated at 16,000 on the ORAC scale, the highest known antioxidant value, more than double the ORAC value of blueberries.

Aronia has been scientifically validated as a preventive and treatment for:

❖ Heart disease

❖ Obesity

❖ Diabetes

❖ Cancer

❖ Alzheimer's disease

❖ Parkinson's disease

❖ Cognitive decline

❖ Depression and anxiety

❖ Liver disease

❖ Exposure to toxic heavy metals

Aronia is now available as a standardized extract, making it more palatable than the tart berries used historically.

Here is a brief capsule of Aronia's scientifically validated properties:

Heart disease

Ohio State University researchers who reviewed several Aronia studies concluded: "Aronia juice may prevent the occurrence of cardiovascular disease, and the phenolic compounds that possess potent antioxidant activity may be the main active components involved."

In addition to its antioxidant and anti-inflammatory properties, numerous studies confirm that Aronia:

❖ Lowers blood pressure by vasodilation

❖ Improves arterial elasticity

❖ Reduces LDL cholesterol

❖ Helps reduce atherosclerotic deposits

❖ Reverses dysbiosis, which has long been connected with cardiovascular disease

Arterial elasticity

In a 2019 British clinical trial published by the prestigious *American Journal of Clinical Nutrition*, researchers attributed the "rich sources of polyphenols" in Aronia berries and extract for the improvement in arterial elasticity in as little at 2 hours after consuming Aronia and continuing through the 12 weeks their male subjects participated in the study.

That research was confirmed in another British study in 2022 that included women in the study group.

Those researchers concluded, "... the present findings suggest that daily consumption of Aronia berry extract led to improvement in arterial function in healthy middle-aged people with a concomitant and related increase in potentially health-promoting bacteria..."

British researchers confirm that Aronia berries help protect against heart disease and attribute that benefit to their positive influences on the gut microbiome.

Prevention of cardiometabolic diseases

Danish researchers looked at 17 published studies on Aronia and made some interesting conclusions:

"*Aronia melanocarpa* is rich in polyphenols and compared to berries of other plants, its berries have the highest concentrations. Due to the high polyphenol content, Aronia melanocarpa may be effective in the treatment and prevention of cardiometabolic diseases and related risk factors. Interestingly, no studies have reported adverse effects of *Aronia melanocarpa* consumption."

Researchers at Tennessee's Franklin School of Integrative Health Sciences concluded that Aronia is an effective way to lower blood pressure and cholesterol in people over 50.

Cardioprotective

Serbian researchers found Aronia supplements improved protection against cardiovascular disease in former smokers.

Type 2 diabetes, obesity, and metabolic syndrome

Since type 2 diabetes and heart disease often go hand-in-hand, Aronia's cardioprotective properties have been validated to extend to diabetes, obesity, and metabolic syndrome.

Improved glucose tolerance

Russo/Serbian animal studies show that Aronia extract supplementation improved glucose tolerance, "significantly" lowered BMI, and lowered insulin concentration in oral glucose tolerance tests. Type 2 diabetes research using an animal model showed not only did Aronia extract reduce insulin resistance and aid in controlling blood sugar levels, but it also promoted weight loss and reduced the risk for fat accumulation in the arteries.

In humans, Bulgarian researchers found that Aronia significantly lowered fasting blood sugars and helped control blood sugars over three months, reducing HbA1c levels from 9.39 to 7.39.

Antioxidant effects

One of the most interesting recent studies was published in the *Journal of Medicinal Food* in 2021 and concluded that Aronia berry extract lessened the inflammatory effects of a high-fat/high-sugar diet. Researchers credit anthocyanin, a polyphenol found in Aronia berry extract, for reducing inflammation, neutralizing free radicals and helping control blood sugar.

Polish scientists found that an extract of Aronia berries increased glutathione levels, the antioxidant polyphenol flavonoid that is perhaps the most potent antioxidant in cells. It's the gatekeeper blocking free radical oxygen molecules, inflammatory markers, xenobiotics and the downstream diseases that accompany them.

Other Polish research suggests that Aronia can help prevent and treat xenobiotic-caused liver damage due to

FOR HEALTHCARE PROFESSIONALS 75

high lipids. Other research confirms Aronia can reduce liver inflammation in non-alcoholic fatty liver disease.

Anti-obesity

One pivotal Japanese animal study confirmed Aronia's glucose-controlling benefits and added a truly important element: Aronia helps reduce belly fat.

We know that abdominal fat can nearly double the risk of dying prematurely, according to a study of more than 350,000 European men and women published in *The New England Journal of Medicine*.

Serbian researchers found that Aronia supplementation reduced waist circumference in postmenopausal women who were morbidly obese.

Cancer

Aronia's polyphenolic compounds and antioxidant, xenobiotic, and epigenetic properties are essential to its anticancer benefits. I have personally conducted research on Aronia extract and found impressive results, primarily against colon cancer, but other research confirms its value against other types of cancer.

Cell proliferation and apoptosis

That pivotal 2022 study from Ohio State cites previous research confirming Aronia's effectiveness against human breast, cervical, colon, glioblastoma, liver, leukemia, and lung cancer, crediting the polyphenols procyanidin, anthocyanin, cyanidin glycosides, caffeic and chlorogenic acids for restoring healthy cellular replication.

Specifically, the Ohio State study credits Aronia berries for selectively targeting colon cancer cells while protecting normal colon cells, a major advance since cancer treatment often damages healthy cells. They also found that Aronia extracts have a unique ability to help overcome chemoresistance, making chemotherapy drugs and radiation more effective at lower dosages while protecting healthy tissue.

British researchers confirm that Aronia reinstates apoptosis, restoring the natural life cycle of cells and their replacement with identical healthy cells.

Overcoming chemoresistance

The Ohio State study also confirms that gemcitabine, a chemotherapy drug, proved more effective against usually deadly pancreatic cancer when combined with Aronia berries. Italian researchers found that the chlorogenic acid abundant in Aronia can work synergistically to improve the effectiveness of doxorubicin, a chemotherapy drug used to treat several types of cancer.

Metastasis and stem cell proliferation

Korean researchers tracked Aronia's ability to knock out breast cancer stem cells, and French research shows that Aronia treatment kills embryonic cancer stem cells and restores normal cell reproduction.

Aronia berries hold a rare place in the plant world because of their ability to regulate rogue genes and restore them to their normal state.

A 2021 study by a consortium of researchers from several countries, including the United States, confirmed

Aronia's ability to restore epigenetic normalcy in over-weight women with heart disease. A German study confirmed that drinking an Aronia juice extract for just four weeks helped repair frayed or broken DNA strands in healthy men.

Neuroprotection

Aronia has the unique ability to cross the blood-brain barrier, opening the door to protecting the brain from dementia and Alzheimer's disease, Parkinson's disease, and a variety of other neurodegenerative disorders.

Aronia is also a key element in protecting neurons (brain and nervous system cells) from deteriorating or dying due to oxidative stress.

A 2022 animal study found that Aronia improves memory and protects brain cells from beta-amyloid plaque. The antioxidant anthocyanin polyphenols found in abundance in Aronia are credited with improving memory and other neuroprotective benefits.

Researchers at the University of Nebraska determined that Aronia extracts protect brain cells from death or damage caused by inflammation and free radical oxygen molecules. Quite specifically, they found that Aronia's xenobiotic benefits protect brain cells that have been damaged by exposure to the herbicide paraquat, which is known to cause Parkinson's disease.

Dutch research confirms that six months of Aronia extract supplement slowed cognitive decline in people who were at high risk of mental deterioration and worsening neurological diseases.

Other studies have confirmed Aronia's protective effects against the "normal" cognitive decline associated with aging, especially with overweight men over 60.

And Serbian scientists found that those anthocyanins relieved anxiety and stress in lab animals.

Hepatoprotective

Fibrosis, the accumulation of scar tissue in the liver, is caused by inflammation linked with alcoholism, chronic hepatitis, and nonalcoholic fatty liver disease.

Korean researchers found that Aronia helps reverse non-alcoholic fatty liver disease and improves the liver's ability to process fats. Additional research using an animal model confirms that Aronia can reverse fibrosis and help restore the balanced ecosystem of gut microbes that are commonly unbalanced in people with liver disease.

Metal detoxification

Polish researchers found Aronia protects the body against cadmium poisoning caused by cigarette smoke, exposure to batteries, lead, and a variety of foods grown in contaminated soil. The human body has great difficulty removing the xenobiotic toxic heavy metal, so it generally accumulates in the kidneys, where it can cause cancer.

Several studies now confirm that Aronia helps activate the body's natural antioxidant defenses to chelate toxic metals like cadmium while protecting the body's vital zinc and copper balances at moderate doses.

Anti-aging

It goes without saying that preventing and controlling the risk factors for diabetes, heart disease, cancer and other chronic diseases of aging contribute to a longer, healthier life. However, there are studies that show that people taking Aronia were far less likely to die of any cause than those who did not take it.

It might even extend to human lives. For example, Korean researchers who tested Aronia on fruit flies found that Aronia supplementation extended the fruit flies' lifespan by an impressive 10%.

Geroprotective effects

Russian researchers call Aronia a "geroprotector," meaning it affects the root causes of aging (inflammation, oxidation and xenobiotics) and age-related diseases.

They credited Aronia's abundance of polyphenols for "The geroprotective properties," including the following effects:

1. lifespan extension in model organisms,

2. amelioration of the biomarkers of aging,

3. low toxicity,

4. minimal risk for adverse events,

5. improvement of the quality of life,

6. evolutionarily conserved mechanisms,

7. reproducibility on different models,

8. prevention of age-associated diseases,

9. increased resistance to environmental stress factors."

French Grape Seed Extract

I strongly recommend combining Aronia extract with French grape seed extract (FGSE), a potent polyphenol, for a synergistic effect.

Aronia's wealth of anthocyanins combines, complements, and even escalates the potent health benefits of FGSE oligomeric proanthocyanidins.

References

Chapter 2: Inflammation: The Good, the Bad and the Ugly

Pahwa, Goyal et al. Chronic inflammation: *StatPearls* [Internet]. Treasure Island (FL): StatPearls Publishing; 2024 Jan–2023 Aug 7.

Morey JN, Boggero IA et al. Current directions in stress and human immune function. *Curr Opin Psychol.* 2015 Oct 1; 5: 13–17.

Chapter 3: Oxidation: Inflammation's Evil Twin

Ren Y, Tyler F et al. Potential benefits of black chokeberry (*aronia melanocarpa*) fruits and their constituents in improving human health. *Molecules.* 2022 Nov 13;27(22):7823.

Chapter 4: Xenobiotics: Our Toxic World

Patterson AD, Gonzalez FJ et al. Xenobiotic metabolism–a view through the metabolometer. *Chem Res Toxicol.* 2010;23(5):851–860.

Srinivas R, Vasudeva M S et al. Xenobiotics in health and disease: the two sides of a coin: a clinician's perspective. *Open Acc J of Toxicol.* 2020;4(4):555641.

Rasmussen SL, Pertoldi C et al. A review of the occurrence of metals and xenobiotics in European hedgehogs (*Erinaceus europaeus*). *Animals (Basel).* 2024 Jan 11;14(2);232.

Stefanac T, Grgas D et al. Xenobiotics—Division and methods of detection: a review. *J Xenobiot.* 2021 Oct 26;11(4):130–141.

Wang YU, Qian H et al. Phthalates and their impacts on human health. *Healthcare (Basel).* 2021 May;9(5):605

Borowska S, Brzóska MM. Chokeberries (*Aronia melanocarpa*) and their products as a possible means for the prevention and treatment of noncommunicable diseases and unfavorable health effects due to exposure to xenobiotics. *Compr Rev Food Sci Food Saf.* 2016 Nov;15(6):982–1017.

Olas B, Kedzierska M et al. Effects of polyphenol-rich extract from berries of *Aronia melanocarpa* on the markers of oxidative stress and blood platelet activation. *Platelets.* 2010;21(4):274–81.

Moskaug JØ, Carlsen H et al. Polyphenols and glutathione synthesis regulation. *Am J Clin Nutr.* 2005 Jan;81(1 Suppl):277S–283S.

Chong JW, Kim JE et al. Eight-week supplementation of Aronia berry extract promoted the glutathione defence system against acute aerobic exercise-induced oxidative load immediately and 30 min post-exercise in healthy adults: a double-blind, randomised controlled trial. *J Hum Nutr Diet.* 2023 Aug;36(4):1589–1599.

Zhang Y, Zhao Y et al. Chokeberry (*Aronia melanocarpa*) as a new functional food relationship with health: an overview. *J Future Foods.* 2021 Dec;1(2):168–178.

Stojkovic L, Zec M et al. Polyphenol-rich *Aronia melanocarpa* juice consumption affects *line-1* dna methylation in peripheral blood leukocytes in dyslipidemic women. *Front Nutr.* 2021; 8: 689055.

Chapter 5: A Home Run!

Rahmann MM, Islam F et al. The gut microbiota (microbiome) in cardiovascular disease and its therapeutic regulation. *Front Cell Infect Microbiol.* 2021 June 20;12:903570.

Istas G, Wood E et al. Effects of aronia berry (poly)phenols on vascular function and gut microbiota: a double-blind randomized controlled trial in adult men. *Am J Clin Nutr.* 2019 Aug 1;110(2):316–329.

Le Sayec, Xu Y et al. The effects of Aronia berry (poly)phenol supplementation of arterial function and the gut microbiome in middle-aged men and women: results from a randomized clinical trial. *Clinical Nutriton;* 41: (2022) 2549–2561.

Jakovljevic V, Miliv P et al. Standardized *Aronia melanocarpa* extract as novel supplement against metabolic syndrome: a rat model. *Int J Mol Sci.* 2018 Dec 20;20(1):6.

Chapter 6: Cancer

Kedzierska M, Olas B et al. Effects of the commercial extract of aronia on oxidative stress in blood platelets isolated from breast cancer patients after the surgery and various phases of the chemotherapy. *Fitoterapia.* 2012 Mar;83(2);310–317.

Salzillo A, Ragone A et al. Chlorogenic acid enhances doxorubicin-mediated cytotoxic effect in osteosarcoma cells. *Int J Mol Sci.* 2021 Aug 10;22(16):8586.

Sharif T, Stambouli M et al. The polyphenolic-rich *Aronia melanocarpa* juice kills teratocarcinomal cancer stem-like cells, but not their differentiated counterparts. *J Funct Foods.* 2013 July;5(3):1244–1252.

Sharif T, Alhosin M et al. *Aronia melanocarpa* juice induces a redox-sensitive p73-related caspase 3-dependent apoptosis in human leukemia cells. *PLoS One.* 2012;7(3):e32526.

Borczak B, Kapusta-Duch et al. Aronia berry extract shows anti-cancer activity in colorectal cancer cells. Poster Presentation 3821: Tuesday, April 18, 2023, 9 a.m. to 12:30 p.m.

Malik M, Zhao C et al. Anthocyanin-rich extract from *Aronia meloncarpa* E induces a cell cycle block in colon cancer but not normal colonic cells. *Nutr Cancer.* 2003;46(2):186–96.

Chapter 7: Heart Protection

Hawkins J, Hires C et al. Daily supplementation with *Aronia melanocarpa* (chokeberry) reduces blood pressure and cholesterol: a meta-analysis of controlled clinical trials. *J Diet Suppl.* 2021;18(5):517–530.

Christiansen CB, Mellbye FB. Effects of *Aronia melanocarpa* on cardiometabolic diseases: a systematic review of quasi-design studies and randomized controlled trials. *Rev Diabet Stud,* 2022 June 30;18(2):76–92.

Buda V, Andor M et al. Cardioprotective effects of cultivated black chokeberries (*aronia* spp.): traditional uses, phytochemistry and therapeutic effects. *Molecules.* 2022 Nov;27(22):7823.

Ren Y, Frank T. et al. Potential benefits of black chokeberry (*aronia melanocarpa*) fruits and their constituents in improving human health. *Molecules.* 2022 Nov 13;27(22):7823.

Mężyńska M, Brzóska MM. Extract from *Aronia melanocarpa* L. berries protects against cadmium-induced lipid peroxidation and oxidative damage to proteins and dna in the liver: a study using a rat model of environmental human exposure to this xenobiotic. *Nutrients.* 2019 Mar 31;11(4):758.

Chapter 8: Anti-Aging and Much More

Yu SY, Kim MB Anthocyanin-rich aronia berry extract mitigates high-fat and high-sucrose diet-induced adipose tissue inflammation by inhibiting nuclear factor-κB activation. *J Med Food.* 2021 Jun;24(6):586–594.

Mu J, Xin G et al. Beneficial effects of *Aronia melanocarpa* berry extract on hepatic insulin resistance in type 2 diabetes mellitus rats. *J Food Sci.* 2020 Apr;85(4):1307–1318.

Simeonov SB, Botushanov NP et al. Effects of *Aronia melanocarpa* juice as part of the dietary regimen in patients with diabetes mellitus. *Folia Med (Plovdiv).* 2002;44(3):20–23.

Pischon T, Boeing H et al. General and abdominal adiposity and risk of death in Europe. *N Engl J Med.* 2008 Nov 13;359(20):2105–2120.

Platonova EY, Shaposhnikov MV et al. Black chokeberry (*Aronia melanocarpa*) extracts in terms of geroprotector criteria. *Trends Food Sci Technol.* 2021 Aug;114:570–584.

Kardum N, Petrovic-Oggiano G. Effects of glucomannan-enriched, aronia juice-based supplement on cellular antioxidant enzymes and membrane lipid status in subjects with abdominal obesity. *ScientificWorldJournal.* 2014;2014:869250.

Handeland M, Grude N et al. Black chokeberry juice (*Aronia melanocarpa*) reduces incidences of urinary tract infection among nursing home residents in the long term—a pilot study. *Nutr Res.* 2014 Jun;34(6):518–525.

Eggers M, Jungke P et al. Antiviral activity of plant juices and green tea against SARS-CoV-2 and influenza virus. *Phytother Res.* 2022 May;36(5):2109–2115.

Wen H, Cui H et al. Isolation of Neuroprotective anthocyanins from black chokeberry (*Aronia melanocarpa*) against amyloid-β-iInduced cognitive impairment. *Foods.* 2020 Dec 29;10(1);63.

Lee HY, Weon JB et al. Neuroprotective effect of *Aronia melanocarpa* extract against glutamate-induced oxidative stress in HT22 cells. *BMC Complement Altern Med.* 2017 Apr 11;17(1):207.

Zhao Y, Liu X et al. *Aronia melanocarpa* polysaccharide ameliorates liver fibrosis through TGF-β1-mediated the activation of PI3K/AKT pathway and modulating gut microbiota. *J Pharmacol Sci.* 2022 Dec;150(4):289–300.

Park CH, Kim JH et al. *Aronia melanocarpa* extract ameliorates hepatic lipid metabolism through PPARγ2 downregulation. *PLoS One.* 2017 Jan 12;12(1);e0169685.

Mężyńska M, Brzóska MM. et al. Extract from *Aronia melanocarpa* L. berries prevents cadmium-induced oxidative stress in the liver: a study in a rat model of low-level and moderate lifetime human exposure to this toxic metal. *Nutrients.* 2019 Jan; 11(1): 21.

Jo AR, Imm JY. Effects of aronia extract on lifespan and age-related oxidative stress in *Drosophila melanogaster. Food Sci Biotechnol.* 2017 Aug 18;26(5):1399–1406.

Chapter 9: Add in French Grape Seed Extract

Malinowska J, Oleszek W et al. The polyphenol-rich extracts from black chokeberry and grape seeds impair changes in the platelet adhesion and aggregation induced by a model of hyperhomocysteinemia. *Eur J Nutr.* 2013 Apr;52(3):1049–1057.

Index

About the Authors

AJAY GOEL

Dynamic and passionate—with a formidable record of patented innovations in cancer care—Ajay Goel, Ph.D., AGAF, is committed to developing better methods for the early detection and precision treatment of cancer. He joined City of Hope in June 2019 as founding chair of the new Department of Molecular Diagnostics and Experimental Therapeutics and founding director of Biotech Innovations at Beckman Research Institute.

A noted expert in gastrointestinal and other cancers, Dr. Goel is currently developing early detection blood tests for colon, pancreatic and ovarian cancers—as well as a test for pancreatic cancer that can detect the disease seven years earlier than is now possible. Within the next few years, these tests are expected to become a simple and affordable part of everyone's annual health physical, just like tests for diabetes or cholesterol.

He is also working with genomic-based precision oncology to provide answers to the question: Why do therapies work with some good candidates and not with others?

Dr. Goel was born in India, received his Ph.D. in biophysics from Punjab University, completed his postgraduate work at the University of California, San Diego, and went on to a noteworthy 16-year career at Baylor Scott & White Research Institute in Texas. He has authored more than 300 articles in peer-reviewed international journals and holds more than 30 advanced genomic and transcriptomic international patents.

Dr. Goel is a member of the American Association for Cancer Research and the American Gastroenterology Association and is on the international editorial boards of *World Journal of Gastroenterology* and *World Journal of Gastrointestinal Oncology.* He also performs peer-reviewing activities for almost 50 scientific journals, as well as serves on various grant-funding committees of the National Institutes of Health.

TERRY LEMEROND

Terry Lemerond is a natural health expert with over 50 years of experience. He has owned health food stores, founded dietary supplement companies, and formulated over 400 products.

A much sought-after speaker and accomplished author, Terry shares his wealth of experience and knowledge in health and nutrition through social media, newsletters, podcasts, webinars, and personal speaking engagements. His books include *Seven Keys to Vibrant Health* and the sequel, *Seven Keys to Unlimited Personal Achievement,* and his newest publication, *50+ Natural Health Secrets Proven to Change Your Life.* His continual dedication, energy, and zeal are part of his on-going mission—to improve the health of America.

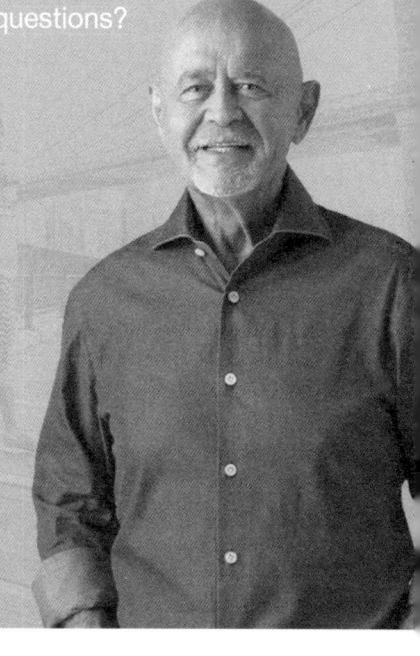

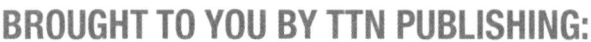
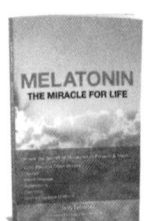
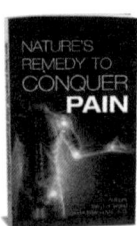
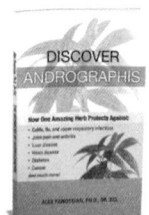
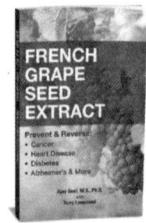
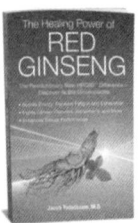
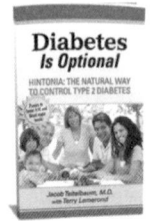
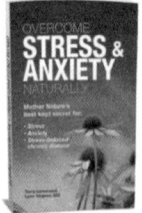
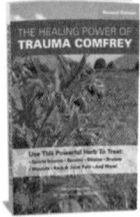
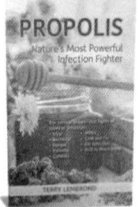